Weight Loss Meditation

*Guided Meditation to Lose Weight and
Burn Fat
Lean in a few steps
Meditations, Motivation Manifestation,
Mini Habits and More*

Jennifer White

Table of Contents

The information in the following pages is broadly considered a truthful and accurate account of facts and as such, any inattention, use, or misuse of the information in question by the reader will render any resulting actions solely under their purview.

There are no scenarios in which the publisher or the original author of this work can be in any fashion deemed liable for any hardship or damages that may befall them after undertaking information described herein.

Additionally, the information in the following pages is intended only for informational purposes and should thus be thought of as universal. As befitting its nature, it is presented without assurance regarding its prolonged validity or interim quality. Trademarks that are mentioned are done without written consent and can in no way be considered an endorsement from the trademark holder.

Introduction

Weight reduction plans are intended to change the diet and mentality of individuals who can lose weight. This overall improvement in behavior and attitude increases the impact of workouts clubbed with good practices.

If you want to be slim and think this is something you cannot do in this life, then you need to change your attitude entirely. While all weight-loss strategies have existed, integrating, and putting all those strategies into a cohesive plan to reduce weight and get a lean and healthy body is something that takes a lot of expertise.

There are some psychological studies which suggest that it takes longer and is more difficult when women lose weight compared to men. Researchers believe body appearance and figure have a more significant effect on women's emotions and values. There are some alternative methods to fast weight loss for women, which can supplement standard weight loss programs.

If you want to remain alive, keep fit because you are likely to run into medical complications with age if you let yourself packing on the pounds.

Just giving yourself go 20 pounds past your target weight makes you vulnerable to developing all manner of potentially harmful diseases such as high blood pressure, diabetes, heart attacks and different forms of cancer.

While most people are aware of the risks for their safety of carrying on extra weight, somehow do not have the will power to do anything about it. Exercising and dieting are items to which people with overweight appear to be allergic.

Chapter 1: Guided Meditation for Weight Loss

Meditation exercise 1: Release of bad habits

Concentrate on your back now and notice how you feel in the bed or chair you are sitting in. Take a deep breath and let your stress leave your body.

Now focus on your neck. Observe how your neck is joined to your shoulders. Lift your shoulders slowly. Breathe in slowly and release it.

Feel how your shoulders loosen. Lift your shoulders again a little bit then let them relax.

Observe how your neck muscles are tensing and how much pressure it has. Breathe in and breathe out slowly.

Release the pressure in your neck and notice how the stress is leaving your body. Repeat the whole exercise from the beginning. Observe your back. Notice all the stress and let it go with a profound breath. Focus on your shoulders and neck again.

Lift up your shoulders and hold it for some moments, then release your shoulders again and let all the stress go away. Sense how the stress is going away.

Now, focus your attention to your back. Feel how comfortable it is. Focus on your whole body. While breathing in, let relaxation come, and while you are breathing out, let frustration leave your body. Notice how much you are relaxed.

Concentrate on your inner self. Breathe slowly in and release it. Calm your mind. Observe your thoughts. Do not go with them because your aim is to observe them and not to be involved. It is time to let go of your overweight self that you are not feeling good about.

It is like your body is wearing a bigger, heavier top at this point in your life.

Imagine stepping out of it and laying it on an imaginary chair facing you.

Now tell yourself to let go of these old, established eating and behavioral patterns.

Imagine that all your old, fixed patterns and all the obstacles that prevent you from achieving your desired weight are exiting your body, soul, and spirit with each breath.

Know that your soul is perfect as it is, and all you want is for everything that pulls away to leave.

With every breath, let your old beliefs go, as you are creating more and more space for something new.

After spending a few minutes with this, imagine that every time you breathe in, you are inhaling prana, the life energy of the universe, shining in gold.

In this life force you will find everything you need and desire: a healthy, muscular body, a self that loves itself in all circumstances, a hand that puts enough nutritious food on the table, a strong voice to say no to sabotaging your diet, a head that can say no to those who are trying to distract you from your ideas and goals.

With each breath, you absorb these positive images and emotions.

See in front of you exactly what your life would be like if you got everything you wanted. Release your old self and start becoming your new self.

Gradually restore your breathing to regular breathing. Feel the solid ground beneath you, open your eyes, and return to your everyday state of consciousness.

Meditation exercise 2: Forgiving yourself

Sit comfortably. Do not cross your feet because this will lock you away from the desired experience. Hold your hands together to connect your logical brain hemisphere with your instinct. Relax your muscles, close your eyes.

Imagine a staircase in front of you! Descend it, counting down from ten to one.

You reached and found a door at the bottom of the stairs. Open the door. There is a meadow in front of us. Let us see if it has grass, if so, if it has flowers, what color, whether there is a bush or tree, and describe what you see in the distance.

Find the path covered with white stones and start walking on it.

Feel the power of the Earth flowing through your soles, the breeze stroking your skin, the warmth of the sun radiating toward you. Feel the harmony of the elements and your state of well-being.

From the left side, you hear the rattle of the stream. Walk down to the shore. This water of life comes from the throne of God. Take it with your palms and drink three sips and notice how it tastes.

If you want, you can wash yourself in it. Keep walking. Feel the power of the Earth flowing through your soles, the breeze stroking your skin, the warmth of the sun radiating toward you. Feel the harmony of the elements and your state of wellbeing.

In the distance, you see an ancient tree with many branches. This is the Tree of Life.

Take a leaf from it, chew it, and note its taste.

You continue walking along the white gravel path. Feel the power of the Earth flowing through your soles, the breeze stroking your skin, the warmth of the sun radiating toward you. Feel the harmony of the elements and your state of wellbeing. You have arrived at the Lake of Conscience, no one in this lake sinks. Rest on the water and think that all the emotions and thoughts you no longer need (anger, fear, horror, hopelessness, pain, sorrow, anxiety, annoyance, self-blame, superiority, self-pity, and guilt) pass through your skin and you purify them by the magical power of water. And you see that the water around you is full of gray and black globules that are slowly recovering the turquoise-green color of the water. You think once again of all the emotions and thoughts you no longer need (anger, fear, horror, hopelessness, pain, sorrow, anxiety, annoyance, self-blame, superiority, self-pity, guilt) and they pass through your skin and you purify them by the magical power of water. You see that the water around you is full of gray and black globules that are slowly obscuring the turquoise-green color of the water. And once again, think of all the emotions and thoughts you no longer need (anger, fear, horror, hopelessness, pain, sorrow, anxiety, annoyance, self-blame, superiority, self-pity, guilt) as they pass through your skin, you purify them by the magical power of water. And you once again see that the water around you is full of gray and black globules that are slowly obscuring the turquoise-green color of the water.

You feel the power of the water, the power of the Earth, the breeze of your skin, the radiance of the sun warming you, the harmony of the elements, the feeling of well-being.

You ask your magical horse to come for you. You love your horse, you pamper it, and let it caress you too. You bounce on its back and head to God's Grad. In the air, you fly together, become one being. You have arrived. Ask your horse to wait.

You grow wings, and you fly toward the Trinity. You bow your head and apologize for all the sins you have committed against your body. You apologize for all the sins you have committed against your soul.

You apologize for all the sins you committed against your spirit. You wait for the angels to give you the gifts that help you. If you cannot see yourself receive one, it means you do not need one yet.

If you did, open it, and look inside. Give thanks that you could be here. Get back on your horse and fly back to the meadow.

———

Find the white gravel path and head back down to the door to your stairs. Look at the grass in the meadow. Notice if there are any flowers. If so, describe the colors, any bush or tree, and whatever you see in the distance. Feel the power of the Earth flowing through your soles, the breeze stroking your skin, the warmth of the sun radiating toward you. Feel the harmony of the elements and your state of wellbeing. You arrive at the door, open it, and head up the stairs. Count from one to ten. You are back, move your fingers slowly, open your eyes.

Meditation exercise 3: Weight loss

Sit comfortably. Relax your muscles, close your eyes. Breathe in and breathe out. Do not cross your feet because this will lock you away from the desired experience. Hold your hands together to connect your logical brain hemisphere with your instinct.
Concentrate on your back now and notice how you feel in the bed or chair you are sitting in.
Take a deep breath and let your stress leave your body. Now focus on your neck.
Observe how your neck is joined to your shoulders. Lift your shoulders slowly. Breathe in slowly and release it.

Feel how your shoulders loosen. Lift your shoulders again a little bit then let them relax. Observe how your neck muscles are tensing and how much pressure it has. Breathe in and breathe out slowly. Release the pressure in your neck and notice how the stress is leaving your body. Repeat the whole exercise from the beginning. Observe your back. Notice all the stress and let it go with a profound breath. Focus on your shoulders and neck again. Lift up your shoulders and hold it for some moments, then release your shoulders again and let all the stress go away. Sense how the stress is going away. Now, place your attention to your back. Feel how comfortable it is. Focus on your whole body. While breathing in, let relaxation come in, and while you are breathing out, let frustration leave your body. Notice how much you are relaxed.

Concentrate on your inner self. Breathe slowly and release it. Calm down your mind. Observe your thoughts. Do not go with them because your aim is to observe them and not to be involved.

It is time to let go of your overweight self that you are not feeling good about.

Imagine yourself as you are now. See yourself in every detail.

Describe your hair, the color of your clothes, your eyes. See your face, your nose, your mouth. Set aside this image for a moment. Now imagine yourself as you would like to be in the future. See yourself in every detail. Describe your hair, the color of your clothes, your eyes. See your face, your nose, your mouth. Imagine that your new self-approaches your present self and pampers it. See that your new self-hugs your present self. Feel the love that is spread in the air. Now see that your present self leaves the scene and your new self takes its place. See and feel how happy and satisfied you are.

You believe that you can become this beautiful new self. You breathe in this image and place it in your soul. This image will be always with you and flow through your whole body. You want to be this new self. You can be this new self.

After spending a few minutes with this, imagine that every time you breathe in, you are inhaling prana, the life energy of the universe, shining in gold.

In this life force you will find everything you need and desire: a healthy, muscular body, a soul that loves itself in all circumstances, a hand that puts enough nutritious food on the table, a strong voice to say no to sabotaging your diet, a head that can say no to those who are trying to distract you from your ideas and goals. With each breath, you absorb these positive images and emotions.

Chapter 2: How to Use Meditation and Affirmations to Lose Weight

Have you attempted and neglected to get in shape? Assuming this is the case, you realize how troublesome it very well may be to stay with a weight loss program.

What's more, in any event, when you know out how to drop those additional pounds, keeping them off is another fight together.

In any case, you don't need to spend a mind-blowing remainder doing combating with your willpower with an end goal to get and stay thin.

One of the key contrasts between those individuals get more fit and keep it off effectively, and the individuals who don't is that the gathering changes their eating and exercise propensities as well as their mindset.

If your mind isn't your ally, getting more fit will be troublesome or inconceivable because you'll be continually undermining your endeavors.

How about we investigate what's required for the sort of mindset that prompts lasting, sound weight loss.

Persistence

Right off the bat, you should show restraint. The individuals who shed pounds gradually and consistently are well on the way to keep it off.
So, overlook each one of those diet designs that guarantee you can shed 10 pounds or more in seven days—the vast majority of that will be water weight, and will be recovered right when you begin eating ordinarily.
It's just human to need a convenient solution; however, if you need to lose the weight, keep it off and move on without having to battle with your body for an incredible remainder continually, it merits adopting the moderate strategy, since compromising makes weight loss increasingly troublesome and tedious over the long haul.

Adaptability

Adaptability is likewise significant for effective long-haul weight loss. If you make amazingly inflexible guidelines about what you can and can't eat, you may get more fit, yet risks are you'll be hopeless.
You're probably not going to adhere to those principles for an incredible remainder.

What's more, when you have this 'win or bust' sort of mindset, and you disrupt your guidelines even somewhat, it very well may be enticing to go on a hard and fast binge a short time later, because all things considered, you've blitz now!

Then again, if you follow reasonable rules while recognizing that there will be times, (for example, occasions and unique events) when you'll eat food that isn't a piece of your ordinary diet, at that point these 'illegal nourishments' will appear to be less appealing because they're not something that you've restricted from your life forever.

Consistency

Consistency is another piece of a fruitful weight loss mindset.

This may appear to repudiate the above point.

However, it doesn't generally. Interestingly, you eat strongly and follow your activity plan most of the time.

Along these lines, you'll stay away from yo-yo and unfortunate practices, for example, the binge/starve cycle.

It's the moves you make most of the time that will give you the outcomes you are looking for.

When you're focused on making long haul changes in your way of life, instead of searching for a convenient solution, you'll be increasingly spurred to embrace a moderate and adjusted arrangement that you can try reliably.

Self-Love

It is additionally imperative to have an inspirational mentality towards yourself. Presently in case you're similar to a great many people who need to shed pounds, odds are you don't feel generally excellent about your body and appearance.

While you don't need to claim to cherish something that you loathe about yourself, it's likewise significant not to be continually beating yourself up for not being at your objective weight as of now.

In fact, you're one of the infinite individuals who will, in general, overheat because of stress, such self-recriminations will most likely cause you to feel even unhappier and significantly increasingly inclined to overeating—thus the endless loop deteriorates.

So, put forth an attempt to concentrate on those things you do like about yourself, and if you have days where you miss exercises or don't eat just as you'd like, be mindful so as not to blame yourself too brutally. Rather, recognize this is something that happens to everyone, and give a valiant effort to put it behind you and start anew simply. Recall that you don't need to eat or practice flawlessly to shed pounds—you simply need a moderate system that is sufficient.

If you can make these things part of your ordinary mindset, weight loss ought to be simpler. It tends to be fairly testing, particularly in case you're accustomed to having a negative disposition towards yourself and your weight loss endeavors. One thing that can assist you with adopting a progressively empowered mindset all the more effective is to utilize a weight loss meditation recording. If you utilize a quality chronicle that incorporates brainwave entrainment innovation, you can increase simpler access to your subconscious mind and utilize basic procedures, for example, affirmations and perception to reconstruct it with new convictions that work for you as opposed to against you.

Such accounts contain dreary hints of explicit frequencies, which make it simpler for your brain to enter a deeply loose and centered state.

In such express, the subconscious is increasingly open to the proposal, and any affirmation or perception work that you do will be progressively successful.

This is an extraordinary method to assist with changing your mindset from the back to front, regardless of whether you're not knowledgeable about meditation or other mind control procedures.

It's justified even despite the little exertion that it takes to do this, since rolling out positive improvements throughout your life, for example, getting more fit is such a lot simpler when you have your mind on your side.
You must not depend on willpower to battle your self-dangerous inclinations—because those desires aren't there anymore.

Control Your Mind, Visualize Success and Lose Weight Starting Today

Our minds are shelled by a consistent deluge of musings, and barely any individuals know about the negative substance that can torment our considerations.

We may imagine that we are responsible for our contemplations; however, frequently, our considerations are essentially a propensity, and we are willfully ignorant of their substance. To get more fit and to have the option to envision achievement, we have to control our minds and prevent negative contemplations from having a free rule. While not in every case simple, one significant advantage to having the option to envision achievement is that you can supplant negative contemplations with positive ones, increment center, and, subsequently, accomplish a great deal more. Since we are continually overwhelmed with data and thoughts that are consumed actually through our faculties, it is significant that we control the nature of these boosts so we can imagine achievement and accomplish our objectives.

There is no uncertainty that we can become affected by outer sources, and if we are not cautious, we can let those sources shape the way that we think, feel, and act.

With regards to our self-regard, those constant bombardments of pictures of ultra-slender models that are depicted just like the embodiment of magnificence can harm our impression of our self-perception.

We can likewise be influenced by pictures of food bundled as sound yet truth be told, might have minimal nutritious substance inside. Figuring out how to control your mind and envision achievement separately will help guarantee that you adhere to your goals:

To accomplish your objectives, consolidate a portion of the accompanying tips:

- Identify your objectives and set little venturing stones with the goal that you can accomplish longer named objectives all the more promptly.

- Visualize accomplishment as you center around those objectives. Ponder how you are going to feel when you arrive at each venturing stone.

- Eliminate negative musings and dispose of them right away. Trust your intuition.

- Set up a simple to follow wellbeing plan and stick to it. Utilize whatever assets are accessible, for example, photograph magnets, practice DVD's, or a prize framework for when you have made progress.

- Practice meditation every night to feel a natural feeling of internal harmony as you continue with your weight loss plan.

- When allurement sneaks into your mind, oust the contemplations and increment your goals. Use affirmations to help oust diet blues, for example, I can, and I will get thinner. Affirmations help you to retrain your brain positively, and if you can picture accomplishment with them as well, they will be considerably more powerful.

Figuring out how to control your points of view requires some serious energy, however, getting mindful of the sheer volume of negative improvements that barrages you every day will push you not just to teach your mind, increment your inspiration yet permit you to imagine achievement and accomplish it as well.

Weight loss in Google, you'll find unlimited locales on the most proficient method to get more fit, however, more regularly individuals battle with keeping weight off or not restoring the weight in addition to additional!

Tragically craze diets, patterns, and pills typically just give you transitory outcomes. They can make you a yo-yo diet, which regularly causes individuals to feel disappointed. What's more, examine shows that traditional diets frequently lead to low self-regard, uneasiness, and melancholy. These sentiments regularly fuel the choice to pick unfortunate nourishments and the cycle proceeds. So, let me offer it to you straight! I've found in my training that 'what to eat' and 'how you work out' are just little bits of the enormous riddle.

What traditional projects ignore is that you'll confront incalculable snags to effectively embracing another daily schedule, and above all, the most elevated obstruction is regularly ourselves.

Traditional weight loss programs mention to us what we ought to do, which is frequently not supportable, and they once in a while center on how we can change our drawn-out conduct.

With regards to getting thinner, the vast majority of us have concentrated on inappropriate things. We haven't taken a shot at the most significant piece of ourselves, our minds. And afterward, we fault and judge the 'program' or mentor as opposed to peering inside.

Chapter 3: Daily Weight Loss Meditation

Before you can begin using meditations to do things such as help you burn fat, you need to make sure that you set yourself up properly for your meditation sessions.

Each meditation is going to consist of you entering a deep state of relaxation, following a guided hypnosis, and then awakening yourself out of this state of relaxation. If done properly, you will find yourself experiencing the stages of changed mindset and changed behavior that follows the session.

In order to properly set yourself up for a meditation experience, you need to make sure that you have a quiet space where you can engage in your meditation. You want to be as uninterrupted as possible so that you do not stir awake from your meditation session. Aside from having a quiet space, you should also make sure that you are comfortable in the space that you will be in.

For some of the meditations, I will share, you can be lying down or doing this meditation before bed so that the information sinks in as you sleep.

For others, you are going to want to be sitting upright, ideally with your legs crossed on the floor, or with your feet planted on the floor as you sit in a chair. Staying in a sitting position, especially during morning meditations, will help you stay awake and increase your motivation. Laying down during these meditations earlier in the day may result in you draining your energy and feeling completely exhausted, rather than motivated. As a result, you may actually work against what you are trying to achieve.

Each of these meditations is going to involve a visualization practice; however, if you find that visualization is generally difficult for you, you can simply listen. The key here is to make sure that you keep as open of a mind as possible so that you can stay receptive to the information coming through these guided meditations.

Aside from all of the above, listening to low music, using a pillow or a small blanket, and dressing in comfortable loose clothing will all help you have better meditations.

You want to make sure that you make these experiences the best possible so that you look forward to them and regularly engage in them.

As well, the more relaxed and comfortable you are, the more receptive you will be to the information being provided to you within each meditation.

A Simple Daily Weight Loss Meditation

This meditation is an excellent simple meditation for you to use on a daily basis. It is a short meditation that will not take more than about 15 minutes to complete, and it will provide you with excellent motivation to stick to your weight loss regimen every single day. You should schedule time in your morning routine to engage in this simple daily weight loss meditation every single day. You can also complete it periodically throughout the day if you find your motivation dwindling or your mindset regressing. Over time, you should find that using it just once per day is plenty.

Because you are using this meditation in the morning, make sure that you are sitting upright with a straight spine so that you are able to stay engaged and awake throughout the entire meditation.

Laying down or getting too comfortable may result in you feeling more tired, rather than more awake, from your meditation.

Ideally, this meditation should lead to boosted energy as well as improved fat burning abilities within your body.

The Meditation

Start by gently closing your eyes and drawing your attention to your breath. As you do, I want you to track the next five breaths, gently and intentionally lengthening them to help you relax as deeply as you can. With each breath, breathe into the count of five and out to the count of seven. Starting with your next breath in, count one to five, and out, count one to seven. Repeat 3 times.

Now that you are starting to feel more relaxed, I want you to draw your awareness into your body. First, become aware of your feet. Feel your feet relaxing deeply, as you visualize any stress or worry melting away from your feet.

Now, become aware of your legs. Feel any stress or worry melting away from your legs as they begin to relax completely.

Next, become aware of your glutes and pelvis, allowing any stress or worry to simply fade away as they completely relax.

Now, become aware of your entire torso, allowing any stress or worry to melt away from your torso as it relaxes completely. Next, become aware of your shoulders, arms, hands, and fingers. Allow the pressure and distress to melt away from your shoulders, arms, hands, and fingers as they relax completely. Now, let the stress and worry melt away from your neck, head, and face. Feel your neck, head, and face relaxing as any stress or worry melts away completely.

As you deepen into this state of relaxation, I want you to take a moment to visualize the space in front of you. Imagine that in front of you, you are standing there looking back at yourself. See every inch of your body as it is right now standing before you, casually, as you simply observe yourself. While you do, see what parts of your body you want to reduce fat in so that you can create a healthier, stronger body for yourself.

Visualize the fat in these areas of your body, slowly fading away as you begin to carve out a healthier, leaner, and stronger body underneath. Notice how effortlessly this extra fat melts away as you continue to visualize yourself becoming a healthier and more vivacious version of yourself.

Now, I want you to conceive what this healthier, leaner version of yourself would be doing. Visualize yourself going through your typical daily routine, except the perspective of your healthier self. What would you be eating? When and how would you be exercising? What would you spend your time doing? How do you feel about yourself? How different do you feel when you interact with the people around you, such as your family and your co-workers? What does life feel like when you are a healthier, leaner version of you?

Spend several minutes visualizing how different your life is now that your fat has melted away. Feel how natural it is for you to enjoy these healthier foods, and how easy it is for you to moderate your cravings and indulgences when you choose to treat yourself.

Notice how easy it is for you to engage in exercise and how exercise feels enjoyable and like a wonderful hobby, rather than a chore that you have to force yourself to commit to every single day.

Feel yourself genuinely enjoying life far more, all because the unhealthy fats that were weighing you down and disrupting your health have faded away. Notice how easy it was for you to get here, and how easy it is for you to continue to maintain your health and wellness as you continue to choose better and better choices for you and your body.

Feel how much you respect your body when you make these healthier choices, and how much you genuinely care about yourself. Notice how each meal and each exercise feels like an act of self-care, rather than a chore you are forcing yourself to engage in. Feel how good it feels to do something for you for your wellbeing.

When you are ready, take that visualization of yourself and send the image out really far, watching it become nothing more than a spec in your field of awareness. Then, send it out into the ether, trusting that your subconscious mind will hold onto this vision of yourself and work daily on bringing this version of you into your current reality.

Now, awaken back into your body where you sit right now. Feel yourself feeling more motivated, more energized, and more excited about engaging in the activities that are going to improve your health and help you burn your fat. As you prepare to go about your day, hold onto that visualization and those feelings that you had of yourself, and trust that you can have this wonderful experience in your life. You can do it!

Fat Burning Meditation

This fat-burning meditation is a simple 30-minute meditation that is going to allow you to spend time visualizing your fat cells, reducing into smaller and smaller cells until they essentially vanish. Focusing on these types of hypnosis, meditations are said to help direct your subconscious mind on how to interact with your body so that you can begin to have a healthier and healthier body. When you focus on intentionally drawing your subconscious awareness into these activities, it encourages it to continue engaging in these activities on its own, even when you are not engaged in your hypnosis session.

This is a great meditation to engage in during the day anywhere from one to three times per week, or at bedtime. They say that meditating right before you fall asleep can be particularly potent, as you are meditating during a time where your subconscious mind is particularly active, and your conscious mind is already beginning to fall asleep.

During this time, you are most likely to experience the level of relaxation and receptivity that is needed for your subconscious mind to really digest the changes that you are seeking to make within it.

Chapter 4: Mantra and Meditation

A Mantra of all the Meditation Forms

This is the second meditation that you can result in when you are facing difficult times and when the events before you have a lot of pressure in such a way that they can make you break the meditation program that you have already started.

This form of meditation is used widely in many schools of meditation.

When you are doing mantra, you select a certain phrase, and it is known as a mantra.

It is a verbal one, and you repeat these many times. At the moment you are repeating this mantra, you should ensure that you are really aware, and you are alert of the mantra that you are repeating.

It is a normal thing to find that as you repeat this phrase, your thoughts may wander to different directions at times.

When this happens, do not give up but instead smile and tell yourself that this is the nature of human beings and, at this point, come back to your senses and continue with what you were doing.

This meditation can work well when you do it loudly but in a low voice such that it is louder than a whisper so that you ensure that your vocal cords are involved. In several cases, you may notice that this may not be possible to you because you are around people, and there are chances that they might distract you and interrupt what you were doing, making you not concentrate. If you find that you are performing these exercises under such conditions, the best way to do is to say the mantra in silence. Do not confuse this to singing or chanting the phrase, but what you need to do is to speak it and repeat it many times. You do this for the allotted time for the exercise before you start. The right suggestion would be to do this for around fifteen to twenty minutes.

 Note that when you are starting and new to this meditation exercise, you will face various forms of resistance.

One of the resistances that you may experience is when you find that the phrase you choose has various meanings, which may be humorous, and sometimes seeing that the phrase has no meaning.

You may also see that what you are performing seems to be something stupid more than anything else that you have done before.

If this happens when you are doing your meditation, do what you have been doing with the meditations during the time of distraction.

Tell yourself that you have been so ingenious in your life, and you have discovered many great things on your research and wish you would live like this on a daily basis and continue performing your program.

This meditation can be done while walking on a road that you are used to, and you know it is not busy, and chances of being distracted are low.

When you do it while walking, ensure that you will not need to cross on streets where there are vehicles because you do not want to lose your concentration so that you can do it to completion and get the experiences it will come with.

Choosing a path that people use to jog may be okay, but you can also consider doing it while sitting or lying in a comfortable position.

When choosing a particular path, ensure that you are comfortable, and the spine is in a straight way such that there is no contraction in your chest.

When you decide which phrase you will use, stick to it, and make sure that you will not want to change it during the time you are performing your exercise.

After choosing a phrase, do not alter for a fifteen to twenty-minute period and you should use it all along for the entire period you have decided to perform the meditation whether it is five or six weeks. Remember that you have already promised yourself that you will learn how to keep your discipline, and you do not want this to fail. When choosing a particular phrase, ensure that you select one that can make sense, depending on the situation you want to focus on. For instance, in this situation, your goal is to control your life so that you do not find yourself doing things that you did not want to do. What you want is to ensure that you are in charge of everything you do in your life, and you know your destiny. When it comes to choosing a phrase, select on something that is relevant to this situation. Some of the mantras that have been used widely before include "Lord Have Mercy" and "God is good," among others. These mantras used by people before were relevant to the situation they were during that time. But for you, choose something that is relevant at the moment. Some of the phrases you may choose are listed below.

- "I want to control my life."
- "I will love my body and guard it."
- "I take charge of my life."

- "I want to take care and nourish my body in the right way" or something else that you think is relevant to you at the time you are doing this.

The third meditation that you can use when you want to deal with those difficult times when the pressure has mounted so much, and you are just a few seconds to wrecking your program, is using meditation in another meaning.

This time when you perform the meditation, you follow a certain passage or a paragraph that is written and contains the way in which you can solve the issues that you are currently facing.

When doing this, ensure you are slow, and your concentration is as high as you can manage.

You do two things at a time whereby you want to read, and simultaneously you are hearing what you are reading.

As you read the word, also try to hear what it means. Ensure that there is a resonation of the word and has a meaning for you. Be attentive to the passage you are reading and do this as much as you can.

If you are in a point whereby you can read the said passage loud, do it, but if this is not possible for you, depending on the situation you are in, read in a way that your lips are moving as if you are being loud, but make sure that there is no sounding coming from your mouth.

After reading your passage or paragraph slowly, take the time and for a few minutes (like three or four minutes) have no plans.

At this time of no program, ensure that you are in a comfortable physical position and try to get the feelings you experience and what happens. Do the procedure several. After performing the exercise, a number of times, when it is during the time of no plans, try to ask about what you experienced and what you feel at this particular time. You will get your answer by feeling and looking at your inner self. When you decide to use this exercise, add it to the program that you already have.

Ensure that you are disciplined enough to perform it on a daily basis alongside other meditations without fail.

When you do this several times, it becomes easy for you and effective.

Many people have found the next meditation to be effective when they want to deal with 'emergency' issues of pressure build-up in their bodies.

When you discover that the pressures that are building internally and externally in your body may threaten your schedule when it comes to controlling your weight, you can try this form of meditation, which has been useful to many people who have tried it.

Perform the exercise on a regular basis and incorporate it with the other medications that are in your program.

When you have done it for several weeks, you can now decide if you will want to continue with it.

If you think it is something that you will want to continue, choose a time that you will be doing it, and it has to be particular.

Do it consistently for the time you decide, and you can always consider it when you find that you are about to experience a pressure build-up.

First, make sure that you are comfortable, and before starting, consider doing some centering.

You could choose contemplation, breath counting, or the Circle of Light.

Now think of your mind as having a white screen for movies and do your visualization.

After you do this, imagine a movie that will appear on the screen after a few minutes showing after three months how your life will be as long as you can take control of it right now.

As you visualize this, ensure that you are realistic since this is not a form of a win that comes like a lottery.

The scent that you visualize on the screen is you after the few months when you will have attained the weight that you desire according to your body if you concentrate on the program to achieve your goal.

If you can control yourself, you will have achieved not only your weight desire, but also you will be in control of the other aspects of your life, and you will upgrade your life close to what you desire it to be.

Picture how your life will be on the screen though it may take time to see this picture; you need to wait and be patient.

You need to be gentle and wait until the screen appears, so you should wait for its development in about fifteen minutes.

You can repeat the procedure the following day, staying with the same picture and gathering the details.

In addition, during another day of the days, you can keep picturing how your life would be if you were disciplined enough to stay in control of your life and not let yourself be swayed by other distractions along your way. After a period of like one week, see the results, and decide whether this is something you would like to continue with or not.

Chapter 5: Repetition of a Mantra

What are Mantras—How and for What Can We Use Them?

There are a lot of anxiety-inducing situations every day—an important job interview, asking the boss for a pay raise, giving a lecture in front of a bunch of people, and so on. Calm breathing often turns out to be insufficient, especially in a stressful emergency situation. In this case, we need to apply another approach: the method of mantra.

10 Essentials You Need to Know About Mantras

1. The hidden possibilities of mantras
The strength of mantras honed by ancient Indian sages over many decades is concentrated, even in their ability to influence the physical level. "Mantras are like different doors that lead to the same end: each mantra is unique and thus leads to the same wisdom: to recognize that everything is one. That is, every mantra has the potential to unleash the veil of illusion and dispel the darkness."
(Deva Premal).

---

2. The language of mantras and their meanings

The language of mantras is Sanskrit, which is no longer considered a living language on the planet, but it is called the 'mother tongue.'

We all relate to this in the same way as our language is a cellular language, a code that we understand at a very deep level.

It vibrates in us something that no other language or sound can.

It is a universal, cellular voice that unites us, no matter our belief system, our nationality, and our religion. You can find translated mantras, but the sounds themselves are sufficient to bring about the beneficial effects. Mantras contain deep, concentrated wisdom, meaning much more than the sum of individual words. It is, hence, almost impossible to translate them accurately without losing some deeper meaning. Therefore, let us consider the translation as a guide and let the mantras work on their own.

3. The power of intention

As something is necessarily lost in the true meaning of translation, the power of our intention is very important.

It is good to have a strong intention and a strong focus inside, but in fact, the effect that the mantra exerts on us is the most important.

This is the true meaning of the mantra to every person who uses it. For each mantra, you will find a phrase called "Inner Focus," which broadly covers the intent of that mantra, but of course, you can also formulate an individual intent.

4. Keep the mantra with you all day

There are countless ways to make mantras part of our lives.

I often carry a mantra with me all day. I would like to encourage you to do so! Carry the mantra with you throughout the day, and whenever you think of it, come back to it, the mantra being the last thing you think of before going to sleep. This is how you can truly commit to a mantra and the specific focus or theme that the mantra represents.

5. It's not necessary to chant the mantras aloud

Mantras do not necessarily have to be heard out loud. Understanding this can be a real breakthrough because it means you could carry the mantra on your own without actually chanting.

So if there is a situation where you feel you need to sing the mantra out loud, concentrate on pushing it inward, carry it with you, and hold it in your being, your mind, your heart—this is the root of mantra practice when we connect with the Spirit.

6. Chant your mantras 108 times
108 is considered a very favorable number in the Vedas.
According to the scriptures, we have 72,000 lines of energy in our body (the nadis), of which there are 108 main channels of energy or major nadi that meet in the sacred heart. When a mantra is chanted 108 times, all energy channels are filled with vibrations of sound.

7. In what position should we mantra?
I recommend a comfortable position for most mantras, one with a straight back; we can relax and yet remain alert.
A position that allows us presence.
Because of this, a lying position is not ideal, it is harder to sing, and we risk falling asleep while doing it.

8. Contemplation

Before each mantra, let's reflect on the topic of that mantra: what does it mean in our lives, do we need it, can we develop in that area, etc.? What can we sacrifice to make this quality more fully manifest in our lives? Thinking through these steps helps to refine our focus further and deepen our practice.

9. The most important "element" of the mantra is silence

Be aware that the most important "element" of the mantra that we reach through it is the silence. This is seemingly a paradoxical thing: the silence after singing is what our soul dives into and is reborn. This silence represents the transcendent, the eternal, the reality, and understanding or achieving this is the ultimate goal of mantra practice.

10. Importance of repetition and practice

The essence of mantra practice is not to get over it quickly and then return to our usual daily routine.
The point is to practice and to integrate the mantras into our lives.
Wherever we go, whatever we do, the mantras accompany us.

This is the benefit of true mantra practice. It helps and supports the path of our lives.

The power of mantras is multiplied by repetition and devotional practice. The more pleasure we can bring into our practice, the more pleasure we get. Like real friends, mantras can help you through times of need and stress.

How Do We Use Mantras in Everyday Life?

The method is simple! We need to talk to ourselves— of course, what we say matters. I may surprise you by saying that it's enough to repeat only three words in every situation when you feel under pressure. These three words are: "I am excited."

Yes, I know it is not what you have expected from me. You may wonder why you should use a statement that is not so 'positive.'

Harvard University published a study in the Journal of Experimental Psychology, in which scientists claim that striving to overcome anxiety may not be the best solution in such situations.

Instead of trying to calm ourselves down, it can be more useful to transform stress into a powerful and positive emotion, such as excitement.

Because positive feelings produce quite similar physical symptoms like anxiety, hence, we wouldn't have great difficulties switching the stress to the excitement. Enthusiasm is a positive emotion; besides, it is easier to cope with. The study also recalls earlier research that mild anxiety can even be a motivator for specific tasks. So, it is worth using the energy generated by stress to increase our efficiency, instead of trying our best to suppress it. To turn fear-based anxiety into a positive feeling, repeat for 60 seconds to yourself, "I am excited." This mantra "redraws" the picture of a stressful situation into something we happen to be waiting for—which is far less exhausting than trying to calm ourselves down. Using different mantras is very important to me, and I use them daily for my meditations or just for relaxation.

You can also use them whenever you are sad, or you don't know where you belong to what you have to do with your life.

They help you to see through and view yourself.

If you have been to a place where people have been singing or chanting, you will know how much power and energy there is in a particular word.

One of the best-known mantras is "Aum" or "Oum."

It is found among Hindus but also in Buddhism. Followers believe this mantra purifies the soul and helps to release negative emotions.

This mantra is also known as a sign of the "quick eye" chakra.

If you want to reach the best result, sing AUM loudly so that its sound vibrates in your ears and soaks your entire body. It will convince your outer sense, give you greater joy and a sense of success.

When singing AUM loudly, "M" should sound at least three times as long as "AU."

When repeating "AUM," imagine that life energy, divine energy flows through you through the crown chakra. The breath that flows through your nose is very limited.

But if you can imagine that there is a large opening at the top of your head, and life energy, cosmic energy is flowing into your body through that opening, you will undoubtedly be able to accelerate the purification of your nature, strengthen your aspiration and hunger for God, Truth, Light, and Salvation.

There are many ways to sing "AUM."

If we repeat "AUM" with the immense power of the soul, then we enter into the cosmic vibration where creation is in perfect harmony.

If the soul completely repeats the "AUM," we become one with the Cosmic Dance; we become one with God the Creator, God the Maintainer, and God the Transformer (Saunders, n.d.).

Chapter 6: How to Practice Everyday

What's the key to taking out weight issues? I'll let you know. The mystery is to demolish the old subconscious squares, produce new idea designs, and fit your cognizant and subconscious mind. Hypnosis can assist you in defeating the difficulties of subconscious squares. You will feel all the more powerful. You will feel in charge.

You will feel sure that you can control your weight with motivation and vitality to adhere to your weight-loss objectives. Hypnosis doesn't have any of the destructive or negative symptoms of diet pills or surgery.

If you pick decent eating and exercise plan and, at that point, reconstruct your mind with the goal that follows, your eating and movement program is not, at this point, hard yet simple, pleasant, and powerful; you will be fruitful.

Have a ton of fun practicing and eating in a solid manner, with the goal that you quit causing self-actuated clash, stress, and demoralization.

You will start normally doing the things that will bolster you in your objective to be sound and get in shape.

You should dispose of the unfortunate idea designs that are making you overweight. These idea designs, which are put away in your subconscious mind, must be supplanted with solid contemplations and sound propensities so you will consequently do what you are required to manage while never mulling over it.

Does this sound confound? It's in reality far less troublesome than you may see. You will require about 10 to 20 minutes per day for a time of at any rate 21 days (the time it takes to build up a propensity). Presently you can have the stuff to program your mind to shed pounds expediently. Hypnosis is one of the most misconstrued yet viable devices for self-change realistic on the planet today.

At the point when you state "hypnosis," a great many people consider Vegas enchantment shows or senseless stage acts. Those individuals in front of an audience were exceptionally picked for their defenselessness to the proposal.

They would do nothing in front of an audience that they would not regularly do.

They simply "don't mind" acting senseless in front of an audience for the consideration they get.

If they don't perform, they realize they will be removed from the stage and back to their seat.

Nothing could be further from reality. Hypnosis is essentially an exceptionally loosened up perspective in which you are increasingly open to proposals.

You ordinarily go into hypnosis commonly during the day.

If significant clinical affiliations have endorsed the utilization of hypnosis to treat malady, envision how incredibly compelling and powerful, it is when treating thought designs that hold up the traffic of the solid body you merit.

The utilization of hypnosis to treat ailment has been around for over 50 years. Indeed, the British Medical Association affirmed the utilization of hypnotherapy in 1955. The American Medical Association affirmed its utilization in 1958.

In a 9-week investigation of three-weight the board gatherings (one utilizing hypnosis and one not utilizing hypnosis), the hypnosis bunch kept on getting brings about the two-year development, while the non-hypnosis bunch demonstrated no further outcomes (Journal of Clinical Psychology, 1985).

In an investigation of 60 ladies, the gatherings utilizing hypnosis lost a normal of 17 pounds, while the non-hypnosis bunch lost a normal of just 5 pounds (Journal of Consulting and Clinical Psychology, 1986).

Different examinations have demonstrated that including hypnosis expanded weight loss by a normal of 97% during treatment, and all the more critically, the viability expanded after treatment by over 146%. It has been demonstrated that hypnosis works surprisingly better after some time (Journal of Consulting and Clinical Psychology, 1996). Indeed, even Newsweek Magazine expressed, "The most effortless approach to get out from under negative behavior patterns is through hypnosis."

If you choose to utilize hypnosis sound tapes or CD's, study the content used to decide whether the proposals bode well for you. Ensure there are no negative proposals.

The mind doesn't hear "no or not," so the accentuation of the recommendation will be I WILL not eat stuffing nourishments. This will give you something contrary to your target. Continuously use recommendations in a positive manner. "I generally eat new nourishments that cause me to feel solid, fulfilled, and sound" is vastly improved.

It is critical to discover how you decipher the proposals. If somebody said, "That entryway ought to be shut," would you get up and close the entryway or simply think, no doubt it most likely ought to be shut and let another person close it. If you got up and shut the entryway, it implies you "surmised" that you should close the entryway. A few people don't care to be determined what to do (direct proposals). You might be increasingly effective in making your sound. You could play a loosening up the sound and afterward peruse or work out your proposals.

The best time for your mind to acknowledge these positive recommendations is in the first part of the day when getting up and in the night prior to hitting the sack. You need a tranquil space where you won't have interfered. If you have a ton of movement in your home, you may need to discover a room where you can close the entryway and be undisturbed. It is for just 10 to 20 minutes. For the vast majority, hypnosis is certifiably not a one-time fix. The impacts of hypnosis are aggregate. The more hypnosis is drilled with post-hypnotic proposals, the more changeless the outcomes become. Not very many individuals can be spellbound once and stopped smoking or get thinner. If they do, they, as a rule, build up another propensity to supplant the one they simply halted. Numerous individuals who quit smoking begin to indulge. They just supplanted one undesirable propensity with another.

If you found the root(s) of the issue, there would be no compelling reason to substitute another propensity. It may demonstrate significant to locate an expert prepared in hypnosis and the difficulties of weight loss. Working with an expert will assist you with comprehension and wipe out the prior programming. Particularly with weight loss, to be compelling, utilize the unwinding and self-hypnosis each morning and evening, changing and culminating your proposals as you get thinner.

You might need to include different destinations after you show up at the weight you are OK with alongside strengthening your good dieting and practicing propensities.

From the start, you should start with the full unwinding, anyway following a week or so, you will have the option to go into the casual modified state effectively by simply checking from 10 to 1. Continuously end your meeting with a proposal that you will feel better, better than anyone might have expected, loose and either alert, perceptive, invigorated, and brimming with vitality for mornings or loose and ready to sleep sufficiently, if hitting the hay around evening time.

Ensure to have a paper and pen close by to record any bits of knowledge that ring a bell while tuning in or perusing your proposals. You may recollect things said to you as a kid that influence your conduct now. For me, I began recollecting a ton of things that were said to me when I was a kid that I never thought annoyed me until I was particularly more seasoned. I simply didn't interface the things I recollected to my conduct. At the point when I remembered, I turned out to be furious. I understood the existence I missed by accepting what these individuals had said or let me know as a kid and strengthened by others and occasions throughout the years.

Weight Loss Affirmations: Are They Enough and How to Practice Them

Weight loss affirmations would one say one is of the numerous everyday affirmations that individuals practice developing themselves, yet would they say they are sufficient without anyone else to cause change and how to do you practice them successfully? This article examines what to incorporate with your positive affirmations for weight loss just as approaches to make them viable.

In the first place, when rehearsing weight loss affirmations or some other self-regard affirmations, recall that you are "working from the back to front." What that implies is that to roll out any improvement in your life, regardless of whether it is centered on your physical body or on your funds, you need to change your mindset and internal mind (your subconscious) before any external switch will appear. While numerous individuals definitely think about this idea, it's not constantly polished so that positive affirmations for weight loss or other self-regard affirmations function as well as possible.

To "be slim," you must, as of now, "accept" that you are dainty, and this is the place the vast majority "tumble off the wagon" and quit doing their everyday affirmations when the external change doesn't come quick enough.

In this way, when you start, choose to give yourself sufficient time to roll out the inward improvement with no "desire" of seeing any external change.

Next, you need to incorporate other every day positive affirmations, for example, self-love affirmations, otherworldly affirmations, and affirmations of confidence and trust.

Why? Since when you are attempting to make a change, particularly when it is about your self-idea, you truly need to "pour on the adoration" to yourself just as ingrain as much "trust" all the while, and in yourself, as could be expected under the circumstances.

Indeed, expanding yourself love and capacity to believe the procedure is basic for any self-affirmations on your run of affirmations to work since when you can build your self-love, you have raised your "vibration" to the degree of affection, which shows things quicker. Additionally, when you have more noteworthy self-love, you are bound to treat yourself distinctively, and before you know it, you've shed pounds easily.

Believing the procedure is additionally significant because the vibration of trust is fundamental for pulling in what you need, which for this situation is to be thin. What's more, coincidentally, when rehearsing weight loss affirmations, it's crucially significant that you not use words, for example, "don't" or "weight" since they center your mind on "what you 'don't' need."

For instance, "I would prefer not to gorge" centers around "overeating."

On the other hand, weight loss affirmations that incorporate words like thin, excellent, fit, and sound are better decisions since they "center" on being "slim, wonderful, fit, and solid."

Affirmation Examples to Use:

- "I love myself unequivocally similarly as I am present."
- "I confide in my procedure in getting increasingly slim."
- "I feel increasingly lovelier consistently."

Inventive Visualization: Once you locate the correct weight loss affirmations that cause you to feel tremendous, get an image of the "ideal for your body" and put it up someplace around your bed so when you get up in the first part of the day, you promptly observe your objective. At that point, close your eyes and truly "feel" like your body resembles that and state your positive affirmations for weight loss, self-love affirmations, affirmations of confidence and trust, and feel appreciative.

Chapter 7: How to Find Motivation

Motivation is one of the most powerful tools in creating permanent change. Your motivation is based on what you believe. And as you are probably aware, belief is scarcely based on your concrete reality. In essence, you believe things because of how you see them, feel them, hear them, smell them and so forth. You can program your mind by taking feelings from one of your experiences and connecting those feelings to a different experience. Let us look at how you can remain motivated to lose weight:

Establish where you are now.

You should take a full-length picture of yourself at the present as a push mechanism from your current position, as well as for comparison later on. Two primary factors are relevant to health. One is whether you like the image you see in the mirror and the second is how you feel. Do you have the energy to do what you wish, and are you feeling strong enough? Explore your reasons for wanting to lose weight. These are what will keep you going even when you do not feel like it.

Assess your eating habits and establish your reasons for overeating or indulging in the wrong foods.

It is assumed that you have the desire to get healthier and lose weight. Here, you state clearly and positively to yourself what you want, and then decide that you will accomplish it with persistence. Use the self-hypnosis routine explained above to drive this point into your subconscious mind.

Determine your motivation for the desired results, and how you will know when you have accomplished the goal. How will you feel, what will you see, and what are you likely to hear when you achieve your goal. Devote the first session of self-hypnosis to making the ultimate decision about your weight. Note that you must never have any doubt in your mind about your challenge to lose weight.

Plan your meals every day. Weigh yourself frequently to monitor your progress as well. However, do not be paranoid about weighing yourself as this can actually negatively affect your progress.

Repeat to yourself every day that you are getting to your ideal weight, that you have developed new, sensible eating habits, and that you are no longer prone to temptation.

Think positively and provide positive affirmations in your self-induced hypnotic state.

Tweak Your Lifestyle.

Every little thing counts. This is an important thing to note if you want to lose weight and slim down. Making a few changes in your regular daily activities can help you burn more calories.

Walk more.

Use the stairs instead of the escalator or elevator if you are just going up or down a floor or two.

Park your car a mile away from your destination and walk the rest of the way. You can also walk briskly to burn more calories.

During your rest day, make it more active by taking your dog for a long walk in the park.

If you need to travel a few blocks, save gas, and avoid traffic by walking.

For greater distances, dust off that old bike and pedal your way to your destination.

Watch how and what you eat.

A big breakfast kicks your body into hyper metabolism mode so you should not skip the first meal of the day.

Brushing after a meal signals your brain that you have finished eating, making you crave less until your next scheduled meal.

If you need to get food from a restaurant, make your order to-go so you will not get tempted by their other offerings.

Plan your meals for the week, so you can count how many calories you are consuming in a day.

Make quick, healthy meals so you save time. There are thousands of recipes out there. Do some research.

Eat at a table, not in your car. Drive-thru food is almost always greasy and full of unhealthy carbohydrates.

Put more leaves, like arugula and alfalfa sprouts on your meals to give you more fiber and make you eat less.

Order the smallest meal size if you really need to eat fast food.

Start your meal with a vegetable salad. Dip the salad into the dressing instead of pouring it on.

For a midnight snack, munch on protein bars or just drink a glass of skim milk.

Eat before you go to the grocery to keep yourself from being tempted by food items that you do not really plan to buy.

Clean out your pantry by taking out food items that will not help you with your fitness goals.

The whole idea in the tweaks mentioned is that you should eat less and move more. You may be able to think of additional tweaks. List them down together with the ones found on this book.

Chapter 8: Developing a Magnificent Self-Esteem

There is mostly a link among weight troubles and low self-esteem.

The reasons can be complex, however people with low shallowness regularly are seeking for consolation or so lace in food. Or, they may lack the discipline needed to appear after themselves and have low shallowness as a result. However, with a little attempt your shallowness can be improved.

In extreme cases, our feelings of self-esteem are formed thru our experiences in childhood. If you were not endorsed to love and respect yourself, then you probably go through low self-esteem. The first rule of getting to know to like and respect yourself is to banish bad self-communication from your vocabulary. Self-criticism is extremely destructive. Your unconscious mind accepts the things you say unconditionally. If you are forever berating yourself for being stupid or foolish, all you are doing is programming yourself to feel that way. Remember, whatever you repeatedly affirm will become self-fulfilling.

After eliminating self-criticism from your inner dialogue, you can learn to love and respect yourself more by focusing on your successes.

Being a good parent to your children is a major success in life and all too often very overlooked. Being kind, loving, compassionate, and generous are also wonderful traits that most people possess. If you have got ever received or executed anything, however small, do not be afraid to praise yourself. Maybe you are doing nicely at work, or you have got executed a private aim.

Always examine what you have completed, acknowledge it, and be happy with yourself. There is nothing wrong with praising and being proud of yourself-—it is something you should embrace. Use the learning to love and

Eliminate Negative Self-Talk

Never ever speak negatively to yourself. This can be so destructive. If you repeat something frequently enough, your unconscious mind will soon accept it as a fact.

So, if you often berate yourself through calling yourself stupid or useless, you are really programming yourself in a totally bad way.

You will then unconsciously respond to that poor programming and in reality, create situations for yourself that make you sense silly or useless. Remember the computer analogy—what your program in is what will come returned out. The human thoughts are exactly like that, so any more you must in no way vocally or internally say (or even think) bad matters approximately yourself. I understand this is not usually clean if you have had a lifetime of bad conditioning and your shallowness is low, however you need to begin fresh from this second on. By reprogramming your "laptop" with effective ideals approximately yourself, over time you may construct more self-belief and vanity. It is a case of "fake it till you make it."

From now on view your errors and mistakes as matters that will educate you something.

Look for the lesson within the error but do no longer punish or berate yourself. Sometimes we analyze the most important lessons via our errors.

The key is to research the lesson, so you do not make the identical mistake once more and hold your self-belief by preserving a wonderful inner dialogue.

Admire yourself approach regularly to help you build your vanity.

Learning to Love and Respect Yourself Technique

LEARN TO LOVE yourself completely, faults and all. When you sincerely love and appreciate yourself, you open yourself up to being loved and revered with the aid of others.

Cultivate the habit of loving yourself via acknowledging your achievements and that specialize in your good points.

Close your eyes, take some deep breaths, and loosen up. Take a few moments to clean away any unwanted mind and allow your thoughts turn out to be still. Then cognizance on all of the little matters that you have done in your lifestyles—any true work you have got done, any accurate friendships you've got cultivated, anything you've got received or been praised for.

Keep your recognition on all of the positives in your lifestyles and experience in reality desirable approximately yourself as you do so.

Enhance or even exaggerate all the feelings and photos via making them big, bright, and very clear. Be pleased with yourself as you try this and repeat the following affirmations:

I love and respect myself.

I am proud of myself.

My vanity is strong.

Repeat the affirmations over and over like a slow mantra, saying the words with total belief and real conviction. This is a good exercise to put very strong feelings into, but make sure you remain deeply relaxed at the same time. Draw these words deep inside you so they really resonate with you.

Continue this technique regularly over a number of days until you feel your self-esteem growing strong. As your self-esteem grows, your desire to improve the quality of your life and be healthy will also grow stronger. When your self-esteem is strong, you will only want to do things that are good for your well-being. You simply will not want to load your body up with fattening food, vegetate in front of the TV every night, or let your body become bloated and out of shape. Instead you will have an inner desire that drives you to make positive changes and improve all aspects of your life. You will also naturally gravitate toward other people who believe in themselves and who have positive aims.

When you build strong self-esteem and a disciplined approach toward, you are eating and exercise habits, it is easy to connect with like-minded people.

Your outer life is often a reflection of your inner thoughts and feelings. So look around you.

If you do not like what you see, make the necessary changes from within and things will soon change around you. You have the free will to make changes, and with a little effort and discipline you will do just that.

If there are issues from your past connected to weight control that have held you back, make a vow to yourself to achieve your weight loss goal in spite of the past. Do not hold on to any anger against those who contributed to your low self-esteem and weight problems. This is a waste of your energy. If you believe other people have caused you to suffer and you hold on to the anger, those same people still have power over you. All this anger does is continue to hold you back.

Use the releasing techniques if you need to let go of any negativity or anger relating to the past. If you need further help, seek out a well-qualified hypnotherapist. When looking for a hypnotherapist for a one-on-one session, call some and find someone you feel snug with. Check that the person's qualifications are from a well-established body and ask for references and proof of insurance if you feel the need. Good therapy is all about dynamics between the therapist and client.

So finding a therapist who inspires you and who can get to the root of any problem is the key to successful therapy.

No matter what, never give up on letting go of negativity and anger because hanging on to negative emotions will only slow your progress. The positive self-image technique will help your self-image. Once again, you are aiming to program your mind with a new belief, which it will automatically respond to.

Positive Self-Image Technique

CLOSE YOUR EYES. Breathe slowly and deeply until your mind is still and you feel very relaxed. Then imagine yourself as you want to be. Create a picture of the perfect you are standing in front of you, full of confidence and self-belief. See the confident way this self-assured you stands and how you hold yourself. Make the picture very positive, bright, and clear.

Now, step into your perfect self and imagine you are looking out through your own eyes. Connect with the positive feelings and notice how good you feel in your perfect self. Amplify the nice emotions and affirm they will stay with you in your everyday lifestyles.

Practice this technique regularly, especially at times when your confidence and self-esteem need a boost.

Chapter 9: Daily Weight Loss Motivation with Mini Habits

Once you have set your plans, written your affirmations, chosen your mantras, begun to practice all the meditation and mindfulness techniques you have learned, what is next? Like anything that you have invested in, it is important to perform maintenance. Being able to reach and stay at your goal weight is only part of the picture because what you are working on is a total lifestyle change.

You want your habits and your decision-making to match the life you want to be living. Let us recap the methods you have learned and show you how to apply them to the future of your new self.

Making Habits Count

We spent a lot of time thinking about the importance of habits. It can be hard to see the behavioral patterns in our lives until we try to change them.

By making a conscious decision to take something that is not conducive to weight loss and replacing it with a habit that it, you have already taken a step towards improvement.

It is said that no one can change unless they want to change, and that is very true. Habits are present in every aspect of our lives, from hygiene routines to how we perform our tasks at work. Habits are what make us drive with our hands on the wheel in a certain way or fold our laundry into a certain shape. Your habits surrounding food and exercise are the ones that count the most towards weight loss, and unfortunately, they can be among the hardest habits to break and replace. Donuts taste good, and TV is fun to watch.

Once you have established new habits, you will begin to wonder why you did not just do things the new way in the first place. The only thing you have to lose from foregoing a sugary snack is the weight, so keep doing it! You will learn that going for a quick jog before cooking a healthy dinner is more rewarding than being a slug and eating salty takeout. You may also see the added benefit of saving time and money. When you cook for yourself and buy whole ingredients, you can make your own convenience foods. Make salads for the workweek, or blanch raw veggies and freeze them to use instead of canned, salty alternatives.

Habits are the key that can tie all of your other efforts together.

You can make a habit of reading your affirmations and reciting your mantras. You can replace a television or video game habit with exercise and meditation. You can break the habit of eating convenience foods by mindfully making a shopping list. Everything we have talked about in this entire book can be tied back into making, breaking, or replacing a habit.

Using History for the Future

We talked about the history of hypnosis, and how it took some very smart people centuries to work out the details of why the mind-body connection works. Take that knowledge with you, because you can glean a few important pieces of information from what you now know about how hypnosis works.

First, you know that hypnosis and self-hypnosis are based on both science and blind belief. You have to believe that the practice will work in order for it to be productive. While the methods themselves were worked out by scholars and doctors, they are only as successful as the patient or subject believes they will be. These men had belief in themselves that they had discovered a new medical tool, and you have to have faith in yourself to be able to use the methods in this book effectively.

Next, you can take comfort in knowing that the methods of early hypnosis, while speculative, have stood the test of time and continue to evolve and grow.

If things do not work, they are thrown away; if scientific research is unfounded, it is discounted. You can see this evidence in the fact that Mesmer's bequest is long gone, but cognitive behavioral therapy is still a much-used discipline. Hypnosis has developed greatly from its early days, but it is still around.

Lastly, you know that no matter how intelligent you are, it takes a while to figure out new things. The men who pioneered early hypnosis techniques continued to push themselves and their experiments to the limit to discover new things.

They were determined to not give up, and you can encourage yourself the same way. If you plan and it becomes apparent that it is not working, you can always reset yourself, reassess the situation and try again.

It is designed to get you thinking about your own history and how hypnosis can change your life in your own present and future. We hope it sparked your curiosity and gave you pause to think about what brought you to your decision to read this book.

—

Positive Words for a Positive Outcome

Here is just one last reminder to think positive! We talked a lot about the power of positivity and how it can have an impact on everything you do. Words do have a tremendous amount of power, which is why mantras can be so vital to reaching a weight loss goal. When you learn to apply mantras to your goals, you are assigning power to positive words, and when you shun the negativity of others, you are taking the power away from their words. Do not let your life be a power struggle. Use strong, upbeat words to describe yourself. Be sure that if a sentence contains both negative and positive statements, that you phrase your words to frame and emphasize the positive component.

It can be difficult to change your mindset, and it will take work.

But do not get discouraged and do not allow negativity to rent any space in your brain. Every day is a new day to wake up and commit to positivity. Think carefully about your words and mind how you speak to and about yourself.

By making a conscious effort to be positive, you will have a great day, and another and another, until being positive becomes your new way of life.

Applying Affirmations Every Day

We cannot stress enough the importance of affirmations. We talked about how writing your own affirmations can be difficult because they require deep introspection. That introspection will serve to make you mentally and emotionally stronger and will give you fuel for your weight-loss fire.

When you take time to write a plan and craft affirmations, you are making a commitment to yourself and your goals. That commitment will be what carries you through the tough times and gets you to the other side. Remember to include all the major elements in your affirmations: what your goal is and why you are setting it, an acknowledgment of the path ahead, pride in yourself for setting the goal, positive self-talk, and a belief statement.

By including these components, you will be able to write an affirmation that you truly believe in. Take the time every day to read or recite your affirmations, and they will become part of who you are and who you aspire to be. This small practice only takes a few minutes of your time and may become the most important words you have ever uttered. Affirmations help us believe in ourselves, even when others might not. Hold tight to them, and they will see you through.

Taking Time for Meditation and Mindfulness

You may be wondering how you are going to make time for all this positivity, habit formation, and affirmation reading. Now we are going to add meditation and mindfulness to the mix. The fact is, we do only have so many hours in the day, but all these elements are so crucial to reaching your goals. So how can you do it? How do you find the time to stick to your plan?

The answer is you make time. When you make a commitment to change yourself, there will be sacrifices. You can try getting up a half-hour early or carving out time after work. If you have a support system around you, ask someone to watch your kids while you go to the gym or take them off the school bus so you can have a few extra minutes to yourself in the afternoon. Where there is a will- and you have the will- there is always a way. You can combine your affirmation and meditation time into your wake up and bedtime routines. Practice mindfulness in the shower. Recite mantras while your grocery shop. You can, and you will find the time. Yes, things like yoga and visualization can be a little time consuming, but the more you practice all your techniques, the more efficient you will become at them.

Be creative about how you spend your time.

If you need to make yourself a loose schedule of when you are going to practice your self-hypnosis methods, it will help you stay on track.

Tying It All Together

By now, you have probably decided what methods you would like to use to aid you on your weight-loss journey.

Any and all of the techniques outlined in this book will be useful tools for you as you move forward. But what happens once you reached your initial goal?

You do not want to slip back into your bad habits or let go of the positivity you have injected into your life. It is important to remember how you arrived at your target weight.

Keep a few old photos around as motivation to stay strong. Continue to make the same good decisions when it comes to food and exercise.

All the methods you used to learn how to lose weight will carry you through the rest of your life, so do not abandon them. If you have worked hard at creating new eating habits, you need to ensure habit permanency by not letting yourself slip back into temptation.

If you decided to lose weight because of health issues, you will have a medical support team that will encourage you to maintain your new lifestyle. Listen to their advice and let yourself be a success story that they tell their colleagues. Be proud of yourself! Your determination and hard work are not to be undermined.

You will also probably be fighting the urge to weigh yourself frequently. Do not give in to this temptation. While it is important to monitor yourself, it is never a good idea to obsess over the scale. You want to continue to keep a positive self-image that is based on how you feel about yourself and not about a number. If you are concerned that you may gain back some weight, continue to weigh yourself once a week and adjust your regimen accordingly. Being able to self-adjust based on your current circumstance is a sign of success. You have done all the hard work; now it is time to use what you have learned to keep your weight in check.

Chapter 10: Overcoming Negative Habits

Fortunately, most of our days have a sort of "groove." Actions in a plan that you perform with little thought are performed almost automatically. Otherwise, our lives become tediously complicated, and we spend a lot of time figuring out how to tie our shoes, prepare our meals, go to work, and more. In this way, we can carry out our daily routines with almost no thought and focus our attention on more demanding activities. Repetitive work in life becomes a habit.

Habits can also be undesirable, and these grooves are deeply rooted in today's patterns. They are against us because they waste our time. For example, if you know that you have a limited amount of time to get to work after waking up in the morning, you'll notice that in the middle of breakfast you'll find the morning paper at the table, pick it up, and usually spend the next hour studying. Spend In the daily news, you could spend a good deal of the rest of your time explaining delays or looking for new jobs.

By the way, in our discussion of habits, we call them "desired" or "undesired" rather than "good" or "bad."

The words "good" and "bad" have moral implications. These mean certain decisions. In the example cited in the paragraph above, reading a newspaper is not morally "bad," but not desirable at this time.

The terms "desired" and "undesirable" are the terms "ego," meaning self-determination, not decisions made externally. As with psychoanalysis, our goal is to push material from the "conscience" camp into the "ego" realm.

In many cases, you may even say that removing unnecessary habits requires more than a simple choice. You may want to consciously discard your habits, but fulfilling a wish is a very different matter. There are several reasons for this. First, habits are inherent in their definition and are deeply rooted in their behavior, so they are reflected without thinking. Just thinking "I don't do" does not necessarily affect us deep enough to stop unwanted behavior.

The longer the habit we have with us, the more often we do it, the more secure it will be, and the harder it will be to wipe it off.

Please quit overeating.

It is not uncommon to start eating without knowing it when already taken a full meal or when absorbed in conversation or work.

Such behaviors are driven into individual behavioral patterns dozens of times a day, daily, and over ten years, actually becoming a second cortex that is as natural as breathing (ironically, overcoming eating habits are becoming increasingly difficult for people). Such habits have physical-neurologic-foundation. The neural pathways in our body can be compared to unpaved roads. This road is smooth before vehicles drive on dirt roads. When a car first rides on the road, its tires leave marks, but the ruts are flat. Rain and wind can easily pass by and smooth the road again. However, after 100 rides with deeper and deeper tires, rain and wind make little impression on the deep ruts. They stay there.

The same applies to people.

To expand the metaphor a little, we were born with a smooth street in our heads. When a young child first buttons a jacket or ties a shoe, the effort is tedious, clumsy, and frustrating.

More trials are needed until the child gets the hang of it, and a successful move becomes a behavioral pattern.

From a physiological point of view, these movement instructions travel along nerve paths to the muscles and back again.

The message is sent to the central nervous system along an afferent pathway.

The "I want to lift my legs" impulse continues in the efferent pathway from the central nervous system to my muscles: "Raise my legs." After a while, such messages are automatically enriched by countless repetitions and automatically sent at electrical speed. Return to the car and the street. Suppose the car decides to avoid a worn groove and take a new path. What is going on the car will go straight back into the old ditch.

Like people trying to get out of old habits, they tend to revert to old habits.

Still, we have not developed any unwanted habits. We learn them, and we can rewind the learning. It can be unconditional. And here, self-hypnosis takes place, pushing the individual out of the established habit gap in a smooth manner of new behavior.

The advantage it offers compared to simple willpower trial and error results from an increase in the state of consciousness that characterizes the state of self-hypnosis.

As a neurological phenomenon in itself, this elevated state of consciousness appears to elevate the individual over behavioral patterns.

A further extension of the unpaved road analogy is that the hovercraft slides a few centimeters above the road, over a rut or habit.

Regardless of the habit of working, the implementation process is the same. Only the verbal implant and the image below are different. To encapsulate the induction process, count one, for one thing, two for two things and count three for three things:

1. Please raise your eyes as high as possible.

2. Still staring, slowly close your eyes and take a deep breath.

3. Exhale, relax your eyes, and float your body.

Then, if time permits, spend a little more time, and introduce yourself to the most comfortable, calm, and pleasant place in your imagination.

Now, when you float deep inside the resting chair, you will feel a little away from your body.

It is another matter, so you can give her instructions on how to behave.

At this point, the specific purpose of self-hypnosis determines the expression and image content of the syllogism.

It provides suggestions for discussing different habits that can be followed as shown or modified as needed.

This strategy can help overcome the habit of overeating.

Overall, we are a country boasting abundant food. Most of us (with the blatant and lamentable exception) have enough money to make sure we are comfortably overeating. As a result, many of us get obese. So, the weight loss business is a big industry. Tablet makers, diet developers, and exercise studios will not confuse customers who want to lose weight.

It is said that every fat person who has a hard time escaping has lost weight. Unfortunately, too often, the lean man spends his life, nevertheless never succeeding in his escape. Despite the image of a funny fat man, everyone rarely enjoys being overweight-most people become unhappy, rarely so confident, and less than confident and ruining their lives. Obesity seems to creep on only some of us, and by the time we notice it, it is a painful habit to overeat or eat, like the excess weight itself. Self-hypnosis can help this lean man release his bond of "too hard" and start a new life. An article in the International Journal of Clinical and Experimental Hypnosis (January 1975) reports on such cases.

Sidney E. and Mitchell P. Pulver cite family doctors study hypnosis in medical and dental practice.

Dr. Roger Bernhardt, while mentioning one of his overweight patients, said that "I brought the patient to the hospital for about a year and a half ago. She went to many doctors to cut back. She said she was rarely leaving home because she was extremely obese; she was relaxing and avoiding people. She came in for £ 380. I started trans in my first session. She continued on a diet and focused on telling her she would like people when she lost weight. She came for the first three or four sessions each week, after which I started teaching her self-hypnosis. Now, this woman lost a total of £ 150, but beyond that, she became another person. She was virtually introverted and rarely came out of her home. She dared to do a part-time job in cosmetics. She hosts a party to show off her cosmetics and hypnotizes herself before the party. She became the state's second-largest saleswoman and earned tens of thousands of dollars."

Instead of reaching for popcorn, potato chips, or peanuts as before, he is now simply focusing on the conversation, the television screen, or the printed page, perhaps except for a glass of water, and I congratulate you on being unfamiliar with anything at the table. The second scene that catches your eye is the dining table.

Do you tend to grab this second loaf? Instead, put your hand on your forehead and remember, "Protect my body." Looking at a cake, a loaf, a potato, or a cake raises the idea, "This is for someone. I'm good enough". With the fork down, take a deep breath and be proud to help one-person flow through the body. Then, imagine a very simple and effective exercise method that simply puts your hand on the edge of the table and pushes it. Better yet, stand up from the chair and leave the table at this point.

Here is another image I would recommend to a self-hypnotist. If you introduce yourself to the screen of this fictional movie, you will find yourself slim. Give yourself the ideal line that you want to see to others. Cut the abdomen and waistline to the desired ratio. Take an imaginary black pencil, sketch the entire picture, and make the lines sharp and solid. Hold photo because you can keep this slender picture, you can lose weight. Then get out of your hypnosis and repeat it regularly every few hours.

Exercise is especially useful during the temptation to be used as a comfortable, calorie-free substitute for fatty snacks or as an additional serving with meals. It would be a good time to practice it just before dinner.

As a complement to this discussion, Dr. Roger Bernhardt, while talking about a patient, wrote:" I would like to touch on one of my patients, Mr. Happiness. (He often said to me, so he has this name in my reasoning: "All I want from life is being happy.") Happiness and I have had many problems together, including my sister's suicide, a heart attack, the end of his business, and the establishment of a new business. But now I am glad to say; he is a happy retired man. He says he comes every 6 to 8 weeks, "to keep the wheels oiled."

Shortly after becoming familiar with hypnosis, I enthusiastically talked to him about it and invited him to use it to treat current problems. He refused. He was afraid of that. After a while, I wrote a small brochure about hypnosis. One day, I handed a copy to Mr. Happiness. A few weeks later, he said, "Oh, that's funny. It's not psychoanalysis, but he says that all you do is ..." and he repeated the steps of the deployment process. It was

"Yes," I replied, "It's a simple one to two. Do you want to do that?"

Again, he refused: "Oh, not me!"

This issue has not been raised again for several months.

It must be mentioned that Mr. Happiness was a fat man and was instructed to lose weight for a heart attack. But what the battle: these potatoes, these rich desserts, and these knives! Then one day, he said to me, "I have done something I recently thought you might be interested in. When I go to bed at night, I count, one, two, three, and I say: I do not eat anything, I just drink grapefruit juice, but I still feel well filled. Patient in the letter: "I only count three.") He then confessed to me that for the last few months, he had done this. He lost weight and felt comfortable doing it. Still, he did not want me to hypnotize him. This is, of course, the beauty of self-hypnosis. He did not have to be hypnotized: he was able to hypnotize himself to accomplish what he wanted. We can do the same. All we need to do is to believe in what we are suggesting to ourselves and feel the power.

Conclusion

Focus on your activities, journalize your progress, thoughts, and move on. Record your success, nature; they will guide you in thinking and solving stress, among other problems. You will not only make an impact on yourself but also on the people around you. Make use of productivity apps on the internet to guide you through.

While writing your journal, consider how you've grown physically, mentally, spiritually, and emotionally or socially. Think about how one area has positively affected other areas. If some things haven't worked out for you, spend some time forgiving other people, forgiving yourself so you can move on. Giving makes living worthwhile.

Albert Einstein believed that a life shared with others is worthy. We have people out there who need you, remember not to hoard your successes. Share your success.

Share your new-found recipes, your attitude, and your habits.

Share what you have learned with others. In all your undertakings, know that you can't change other people but yourself, therefore, be mindful.

Reflect on your changes and put yourself on the back today and every day. Be grateful and live your life as a champion.

Make it a reality on your mind the fact that the journey to a healthy life and weight loss is long and has many challenges. Pieces of Stuff we consider more important in life require our full cooperation towards them. Just because you are facing problems in your weight loss journey, it does not mean that you should stop, instead show and prove to the whole world how good your ability to handle constant challenges is—train your brain to know that eating healthy food together with functional exercises can work miracles. Make it your choice and not something you are forced to do by a third party.

Always tell yourself that weight loss is a long process and not an event.

Take every day of your days to celebrate your achievements because these achievements are what piles up to massive victory.

Make a list of stuff you would like to change when you get healthy, they may be small size-clothes, being able to accumulate enough energy, participating in your most loved sports you have been admiring for a more extended period, feeling self-assured.

Make these tips your number one source of empowerment; you will end up completing your 30 days even without noticing. You have made it, or you are about to make it. The journey has been unbelievable. And by now, you must be having a story to tell. Concentrate on finishing strongly. Keep up the excellent eating design you have adopted. Remember, you are not working on temporary changes but long-term goals. Therefore, lifestyle changes should not be stopped when the weight is lost. Remind yourself always of essential habits that are easier to follow daily. They include trusting yourself and the process by acknowledging that the real change lies in your hands. Stop complacency, arise, walk around for at least thirty minutes away. Your breakfast is the most important meal you deserve. Eat your breakfast like a queen. For each diet you take, add a few proteins and natural fats. Don't let hunger kill you, eat more, but just what is recommended, bring snacks and other meals 3- five times a day. Have more veggies and fruits like 5-6 rounds in 24 hours. Almost 90% of Americans do not receive enough vegetables and fruits to their satisfaction.

Remember, Apple will not make you grow fat.

Lightning Source UK Ltd.
Milton Keynes UK
UKHW022300120421
381888UK00003B/407

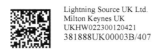

9 781802 081756